Bring On Fitness

About Bring On Fitness

Our passion for fitness gave life to **Bring On Fitness**. We started with the goal of helping as many people as we can. To educate, motivate and to help change peoples lives for the better. Bring On Fitness is not only for the fitness enthusiasts, but also for the beginner. We strongly believe nothing is more important than learning the basics and creating a strong foundation in both nutrition - through meal planning, and in exercise - by following a specific plan. This is just as important for the beginner, as it is for the experienced athlete.

We set high standards for ourselves, the information we share, and the products we carry. Our goal is to provide you with exceptional products that suit your needs and the knowledge and motivation to help you work towards and achieve your health and fitness goals.

Keep up to date by liking us on Facebook and Instagram @bringonfitness

For more check us out at:
https://www.northstarreaders.com/bringonfitness

"Our Mission is to have a positive impact in changing peoples lives. We will deliver the best possible fitness and nutrition solutions that will empower people to achieve their health and fitness goals."

Table of Contents

Bring On Fitness

Introduction

I want to thank you for choosing this book, *'Protein Shakes: Top 50 Protein Shake Recipes for Building Muscle.'*

Many of us want to gain muscle, become lean, build a strong core and lead a healthy life. But the path to a perfectly toned body is one that requires a lot of hard work and restraint. You cannot just build strong muscles by spending hours in the gym, eating a healthy diet goes hand in hand with this.

Getting the right nutrition is extremely important – your diet has to be well-rounded to provide you with all the nutrition that your body needs. If you eat the right kinds of foods that are high in protein, along with exercising consistently, you will be able to get the results you want and build strong muscles.

For those of you who want to take the first step toward building a healthy body, this book is the perfect starting point to make your journey toward muscle-building easier; we have compiled and created 50 protein shake recipes that will help you build strong and healthy muscles. This book contains delicious recipes that will offer you the protein content your body needs.

These shakes are made from a variety of healthy and nutritious ingredients that range from fresh fruit, healthy nuts, wholesome milk varieties, whey protein powders, chocolate and peanut butter to fresh berries. All the ingredients, when blended together in a shake, complete your daily nutritional needs and are also tasty to your palate, making them the perfect kick-start to your day.

These protein shakes can be had pre or post workout, as a breakfast shake, as meal supplements and also as a mid-day snack to satisfy your food cravings. High in energy, these protein shakes will help your body get the right nutrition and the minimal fat and carb content of these shakes will ensure you build strong and lean muscles.

All these recipes come with the actual nutritional and calorie count, so it becomes easy to manage your daily nutrition and calorific needs. So what are you waiting for? Get started with these easy to make, high on taste and nutrition protein shakes and watch your body transform.

Thank you once again for choosing this book – happy reading!

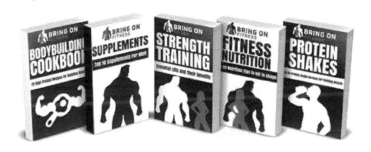

Chapter 1 - Fruit Based Shakes

Muscular Mango

Serves: 2

Nutritional values per serving:

- Calories – 600
- Fat – 4.3 g
- Carbohydrate – 79.5 g
- Protein – 63.5 g

Ingredients:

- 2 cups apple juice, unsweetened
- 4 tablespoons orange juice concentrate
- 1 cup frozen mango
- 4 scoops vanilla protein powder
- 1 cup Greek yogurt
- 1 cup frozen pineapple chunks

Method:

1. Add apple juice, orange juice concentrate, mango, protein powder, yogurt and pineapple into a blender.
2. Blend for 30-40 seconds or until smooth.
3. Pour into tall glasses.
4. Serve with crushed ice.

The Fuzzy Protein Shake

Serves: 2

Nutritional values per serving:

- Calories – 377
- Fat – 4.2 g
- Carbohydrate – 21.3 g
- Protein – 62.7 g

Ingredients:

- 2 cups apple juice, unsweetened
- 1 cup Greek yogurt
- 4 scoops vanilla protein powder
- 1 cup frozen peach

Method:

1. Add apple juice, yogurt, protein powder and peach into a blender.
2. Blend for 30-40 seconds or until smooth.
3. Pour into tall glasses.
4. Serve with crushed ice.

Wild Berry Shake

Serves: 2

Nutritional values per serving:

- Calories – 616
- Fat – 3 g
- Carbohydrate – 79 g
- Protein – 68 g

Ingredients:

- 2 cups raspberries
- 2 cups blueberries
- 2 cups strawberries
- 4 cups fat free milk
- 4 scoops whey protein powder, unflavored
- 2 cups ice

Method:

1. Add all the berries, milk, protein powder and ice into a blender.
2. Blend for 30-40 seconds or until smooth.
3. Pour into tall glasses and serve.

Peaches and Cream Shake

Serves: 2

Nutritional values per serving:

- Calories – 234
- Fat – 5 g
- Carbohydrate – 19 g
- Protein – 27 g

Ingredients:

- 2 scoops vanilla whey protein powder
- 2 whole frozen peaches, deseeded, chopped
- Stevia powder to taste
- 2 cups water
- ¼ cup low fat sour cream

Method:

1. Add protein powder, peach, stevia, water and sour cream into a blender.
2. Blend for 30-40 seconds or until smooth.
3. Pour into tall glasses.
4. Serve with crushed ice.

Honey and Banana Shake

Serves: 2

Nutritional values per serving:

- Calories – 439
- Fat – 7 g
- Carbohydrate – 49 g
- Protein – 45 g

Ingredients:

- 2 scoops vanilla protein powder
- 1 ½ cups nonfat plain Greek yogurt
- 2 teaspoons flaxseed oil
- 2 scoops spirulina
- ¼ cup water
- 2 medium bananas, peeled, sliced
- 4 teaspoons honey

Method:

1. Add protein powder, yogurt, flaxseed oil, spirulina, water, banana and honey into a blender.
2. Blend for 30-40 seconds or until smooth.
3. Pour into tall glasses.
4. Serve with crushed ice.

Tropical Punch Protein Shake

Serves: 2

Nutritional values per serving:

- Calories – 692
- Fat – 50 g
- Carbohydrate – 30 g
- Protein – 30 g

Ingredients:

- ½ cup pineapple chunks
- 6 strawberries, sliced
- 2 ounces water
- 2 scoops vanilla protein powder
- 1 medium banana, peeled, sliced
- 2 cups canned, full fat coconut milk
- 1 cup ice

Method:

1. Add all the fruits, milk, protein powder and water into a blender.
2. Blend for 30-40 seconds or until smooth.
3. Pour into tall glasses.
4. Serve with crushed ice.

Vita-Plum Shake

Serves: 2

Nutritional values per serving:

- Calories – 297
- Fat – 3 g
- Carbohydrate – 17 g
- Protein – 50 g

Ingredients:

- 2 plums, pitted
- 2 cups ice
- 4 scoops vanilla protein powder
- 4 cups water
- Juice of 2 lemons

Method:

1. Add plum, ice, protein powder, water, and lemon juice into a blender.
2. Blend for 30-40 seconds or until smooth.
3. Pour into tall glasses and serve.

Pineapple Power Shake

Serves: 2

Nutritional values per serving:

- Calories – 436
- Fat – 5 g
- Carbohydrate – 69 g
- Protein – 30 g

Ingredients:

- 1 ½ cups strawberries
- 2 cups pineapple juice
- 2 medium bananas, peeled, sliced
- 2 scoops vanilla protein powder
- 2 tablespoons nonfat plain Greek yogurt
- 2 cups ice

Method:

1. Add strawberries, pineapple juice, banana, protein powder, yogurt and ice into a blender.
2. Blend for 30-40 seconds or until smooth.
3. Pour into tall glasses and serve.

Cinnamon Banana Protein Shake

Serves: 4

Nutritional values per serving:

- Calories – 282
- Fat – 6 g
- Carbohydrate – 34 g
- Protein – 25 g

Ingredients:

- 4 small bananas, peeled, sliced, frozen
- ½ cup nonfat plain Greek yogurt
- 2 tablespoons almond butter
- 2 teaspoons pure vanilla extract
- ½ teaspoon freshly grated nutmeg or to taste
- 2 cups cashew milk, unsweetened
- 3 scoops vanilla whey protein powder
- 1 tablespoon raw honey
- 2 teaspoons ground cinnamon

Method:

1. Add almond butter, vanilla extract, nutmeg, cashew milk, honey, cinnamon, banana, protein powder, yogurt and ice into a blender.
2. Blend for 30-40 seconds or until smooth.
3. Pour into tall glasses and serve.

Mango Chili Smoothie

Serves: 4

Nutritional values per serving:

- Calories – 323
- Fat – 8 g
- Carbohydrate – 61 g
- Protein – 6 g

Ingredients:

- 5 cups mango, peeled, deseeded, chopped, frozen
- 4 tablespoons dried goji berries
- 3 cups apple juice, unsweetened
- Juice of 2 limes
- 6 tablespoons hemp seeds
- 2 teaspoons chili powder
- 2 cups water

Method:

1. Add mango, goji berries, apple juice, lime juice, hemp seeds, chili powder and water into the blender.
2. Blend for 30-40 seconds or until smooth.
3. Pour into tall glasses and serve with crushed ice.

Aloha Bliss Pineapple Protein Smoothie

Serves: 6

Nutritional values per serving:

- Calories – 349
- Fat – 5 g
- Carbohydrate – 55 g
- Protein – 27 g

Ingredients:

- 4 scoops vanilla whey protein powder
- 2 mangoes, peeled, deseeded, chopped
- 2 cans (20 ounces each) pineapple chunks in juice
- 2 bananas, peeled, sliced, frozen
- 2 cups light coconut milk
- 2 cups ice cubes
- 2 cups nonfat vanilla Greek yogurt
- 1 cup orange juice, unsweetened

Method:

1. Add whey protein powder, mangoes and pineapple chunks with their own juice, banana, coconut milk, ice, yogurt and orange juice into the blender.
2. Blend for 30-40 seconds or until smooth.
3. Pour into tall glasses and serve.

Chapter 2 - Chocolate, Coffee and Caramel based Shakes

Almond Joy

Serves: 2

Nutritional values per serving:

- Calories – 1042
- Fat – 45 g
- Carbohydrate – 58.8 g
- Protein – 68.8 g

Ingredients:

- 2 cups almond milk, unsweetened
- 4 tablespoons almond butter
- ½ cup shredded coconut
- 4 scoops chocolate protein powder
- 4 tablespoons dark chocolate chips

Method:

1. Add almond milk, almond butter, coconut, protein powder and chocolate chips into a blender.
2. Blend for 30-40 seconds or until smooth.
3. Pour into tall glasses.
4. Serve with crushed ice.

Caramel Coffee

Serves: 2

Nutritional values per serving:

- Calories – 340
- Fat – 6.5 g
- Carbohydrate – 25 g
- Protein – 51 g

Ingredients:

- 2 cups almond milk, unsweetened
- 2 tablespoons instant coffee or to taste
- 4 scoops protein powder
- 2 teaspoons caramel creamer

Method:

1. Add milk, coffee, protein powder and creamer into a blender.
2. Blend for 30-40 seconds or until smooth.
3. Pour into tall glasses.
4. Serve with crushed ice.

Dark Chocolate Banana Shake

Serves: 2

Nutritional values per serving:

- Calories – 565
- Fat – 15.6 g
- Carbohydrate – 58.3 g
- Protein – 54.3 g

Ingredients:

- 2 cups almond milk, unsweetened
- 2 teaspoons cinnamon powder
- 1 banana, peeled, sliced, frozen
- 4 scoops chocolate protein powder
- 4 tablespoons dark chocolate chips

Method:

1. Add almond milk, banana, cinnamon powder, protein powder and chocolate chips into a blender.
2. Blend for 30-40 seconds or until smooth.
3. Pour into tall glasses.
4. Serve with crushed ice.

Rich Shake

Serves: 2

Nutritional values per serving:

- Calories – 591
- Fat – 13 g
- Carbohydrate – 51.7 g
- Protein – 71.3 g

Ingredients:

- 3 cups fat free milk
- 4 tablespoons fat free vanilla yogurt
- 4 tablespoons hazelnut coffee
- 4 scoops chocolate protein powder
- 2 tablespoons peanut butter
- ¼ cup caramel ice cream topping

Method:

1. Add milk, yogurt, coffee, protein powder, peanut butter and caramel ice cream topping into a blender.
2. Blend for 30-40 seconds or until smooth.
3. Pour into tall glasses.
4. Serve with crushed ice.

Vanilla Coffee Shake

Serves: 2

Nutritional values per serving:

- Calories – 482
- Fat – 7 g
- Carbohydrate – 39 g
- Protein – 66 g

Ingredients:

- 3 cups fat free milk
- 4 scoops vanilla protein powder
- 2 cups low fat coffee flavored ice cream

Method:

1. Add milk, protein powder and ice cream into a blender.
2. Blend for 30-40 seconds or until smooth.
3. Pour into tall glasses and serve.

Snickers Mocha

Serves: 2

Nutritional values per serving:

- Calories – 136
- Fat – 4.5 g
- Carbohydrate – 30 g
- Protein – 32 g

Ingredients:

- 1 cup almond milk, unsweetened
- 1 cup cold coffee
- 2 teaspoons butternut flavoring extract
- Ice cubes, as required
- 2 scoops protein powder
- 2 teaspoons sugar free caramel creamer
- ½ - 1 packet chocolate carnation instant breakfast

Method:

1. Add all the ingredients into a blender.
2. Blend for 30-40 seconds or until smooth.
3. Pour into tall glasses and serve.

Chocolate Lovers' Shake

Serves: 2

Nutritional values per serving:

- Calories – 364
- Fat – 17 g
- Carbohydrate – 2 g
- Protein – 51 g

Ingredients:

- 2 teaspoons cocoa powder, unsweetened
- 4 scoops chocolate protein powder
- Stevia powder to taste
- 3 cups water
- ¼ cup low fat sour cream
- 4 teaspoons flaxseed oil

Method:

1. Add cocoa, protein powder, Stevia, water sour cream and flaxseed oil into a blender.
2. Blend for 30-40 seconds or until smooth.
3. Pour into tall glasses.
4. Serve with crushed ice.

Chocolate Peanut Butter

Serves: 2

Nutritional values per serving:

- Calories – 524
- Fat – 25.4 g
- Carbohydrate – 35.5 g
- Protein – 57.1 g

Ingredients:

- 2 ½ cups water
- 2 tablespoons flaxseed meal
- 4 tablespoon heavy whipping cream
- 4 scoops chocolate protein powder
- 2 tablespoons peanut butter
- 2 cups ice cubes

Method:

1. Add water, flaxseed meal, whipping cream, protein powder, peanut butter and ice cubes into a blender.
2. Blend for 30-40 seconds or until smooth.
3. Pour into tall glasses and serve.

Mocha

Serves: 2

Nutritional values per serving:

- Calories – 215
- Fat – 20 g
- Carbohydrate – 36 g
- Protein – 20 g

Ingredients:

- 2 cups hot coffee
- 4 tablespoons honey
- 2 scoops chocolate whey protein powder

Method:

1. Divide the hot coffee equally into 2 mugs.
2. Add 2 tablespoons honey into each mug.
3. Add a scoop of protein powder into each mug.
4. Stir and serve right away.

Chapter 3 - Dessert Protein Shakes

Cheesecake Shake

Serves: 2

Nutritional values per serving:

- Calories – 460
- Fat – 8.9 g
- Carbohydrate – 38.9 g
- Protein – 56.4 g

Ingredients:

- 2 cups almond milk
- 2 ounces cream cheese
- 4 scoops vanilla protein powder
- ½ cup crushed Graham crackers

Method:

1. Add almond milk, cream cheese, protein powder and Graham crackers into a blender.
2. Blend for 30-40 seconds or until smooth.
3. Pour into tall glasses.
4. Serve with crushed ice.

Cinnamon Roll Shake

Serves: 2

Nutritional values per serving:

- Calories – 160
- Fat – 2 g
- Carbohydrate – 11 g
- Protein – 25 g

Ingredients:

- 4 scoops vanilla protein powder
- ½ tablespoon ground cinnamon
- 2 teaspoons butter flavor extract
- 2 cups water
- 2 tablespoons sugar-free vanilla pudding mix
- ½ teaspoon vanilla extract
- 2 cups ice

Method:

1. Add all the ingredients into a blender.
2. Blend for 30-40 seconds or until smooth.
3. Pour into tall glasses and serve.

Apple Crumble Protein Smoothie

Serves: 4

Nutritional values per serving:

- Calories – 228
- Fat – 8 g
- Carbohydrate – 22 g
- Protein – 18 g

Ingredients:

- 2 apples, peeled, chopped
- 2 scoops vanilla whey protein
- ½ cup ground flaxseeds
- 1/8 teaspoon freshly ground nutmeg or to taste
- 3 cups almond milk, unsweetened
- ½ cup old fashioned oats
- ½ teaspoon ground cinnamon

Method:

1. Add apples, whey protein, ground flaxseeds, milk, oats and spices into a blender.
2. Blend for 30-40 seconds or until smooth.
3. Pour into tall glasses and serve with crushed ice.

Cake Batter Protein Shake

Serves: 4

Nutritional values per serving:

- Calories – 259
- Fat – 1 g
- Carbohydrate – 30 g
- Protein – 25 g

Ingredients:

- 2 cups nonfat plain Greek yogurt
- 1 cup almond milk, unsweetened
- 2 cups nonfat whipped topping
- 2 teaspoon vanilla extract
- 2 scoops vanilla whey protein powder
- 2 teaspoons rainbow sprinkles
- 4 tablespoons agave nectar
- 1 cup ice cubes

Method:

1. Add yogurt, almond milk, whipped topping, vanilla, protein powder, agave nectar and ice cubes into a blender.
2. Blend for 30-40 seconds or until smooth.
3. Pour into tall glasses.
4. Sprinkle rainbow sprinkles on top and serve.

Gingerbread Cookie Shake

Serves: 2

Nutritional values per serving:

- Calories – 307
- Fat – 2 g
- Carbohydrate – 34 g
- Protein – 40 g

Ingredients:

- 1 scoop chocolate whey protein powder
- 1 scoop vanilla whey protein powder
- 1 cup nonfat vanilla Greek yogurt
- 1 cup vanilla almond milk, unsweetened
- 1 teaspoon ground cinnamon
- ½ teaspoon ground cloves
- 1 teaspoon ground ginger
- 2 cups ice cubes
- 2 tablespoons blackstrap molasses

Method:

1. Add all the ingredients into a blender.
2. Blend for 30-40 seconds or until smooth.
3. Pour into tall glasses and serve.

Pumpkin Pie Protein Smoothie

Serves: 4

Nutritional values per serving:

- Calories – 201
- Fat – 0 g
- Carbohydrate – 44 g
- Protein – 8 g

Ingredients:

- 2 bananas, peeled, sliced, frozen
- 1 cup skim milk
- 1 cup nonfat vanilla Greek yogurt
- ½ teaspoon pumpkin pie spice
- ½ teaspoon ground cinnamon
- 4 tablespoons pure maple syrup
- 2 cups ice
- 1 1/3 cups pumpkin puree

Method:

1. Add banana, milk, yogurt, spices, maple syrup, ice and pumpkin puree into a blender.
2. Blend for 30-40 seconds or until smooth.
3. Pour into tall glasses and serve.

Peach Cobbler

Serves: 2

Nutritional values per serving:

- Calories – 305
- Fat – 2 g
- Carbohydrate – 49 g
- Protein – 24 g

Ingredients:

- 2 scoops vanilla whey protein powder
- 2 packets Quaker Lower Sugar Maple and Brown Sugar Instant Oatmeal
- 2 cups water
- 1 can sliced peaches in juice, drained

Method:

1. Add all the ingredients into a blender.
2. Blend for 30-40 seconds or until smooth.
3. Pour into tall glasses and serve with crushed ice.

Chocolate Almond Brownie

Serves: 2

Nutritional values per serving:

- Calories – 457
- Fat – 17 g
- Carbohydrate – 41 g
- Protein – 39 g

Ingredients:

- 2 cups fat free milk
- 2 scoops chocolate whey protein
- ½ cups almonds, chopped
- 1 Clif chocolate brownie bar, finely chopped
- Ice cubes, as required

Method:

1. Add milk, whey protein and ice into a blender.
2. Blend for 30-40 seconds or until smooth.
3. Pour into tall glasses.
4. Top with brownie bar pieces and almonds and serve with crushed ice.

Root Beer Float

Serves: 2

Nutritional values per serving:

- Calories – 443
- Fat – 1 g
- Carbohydrate – 61 g
- Protein – 48 g

Ingredients:

- 2 scoops vanilla casein protein
- 2 scoops vanilla whey protein
- 3 cups root beer
- 1 cup fat free vanilla yogurt

Method:

1. Add yogurt into a bowl. Add protein powders, a little at a time and mix well each time.
2. Pour 1 ½ cups root beer into each of 2 large glasses.
3. Divide the yogurt mixture into the glasses, taking care not to stir.
4. Serve right away.

Chapter 4 - Nut Based Shakes

Banana Almond Cream Shake

Serves: 2

Nutritional values per serving:

- Calories – 320
- Fat - 8 g
- Carbohydrate - 32 g
- Protein - 32 g

Ingredients:

- 1 scoop pea protein
- 1 scoop rice protein
- 1 cup skim milk
- 2 bananas, peeled, chopped
- 20 almonds
- 1 cup ice

Method:

1. Add protein powders, milk, banana, almonds and ice into a blender.
2. Blend for 30-40 seconds or until smooth.
3. Pour into tall glasses and serve.

Soy Almond Shake

Serves: 2

Nutritional values per serving:

- Calories – 312
- Fat – 8 g
- Carbohydrate – 26 g
- Protein – 34 g

Ingredients:

- 2 scoops vanilla protein powder
- 2 tablespoons almonds, chopped
- 2 teaspoons vanilla extract
- 2 cups ice
- 2 cups light soy milk
- 2 teaspoons sugar free maple syrup
- 2 tablespoons plain nonfat Greek yogurt

Method:

1. Add all the ingredients into a blender.
2. Blend for 30-40 seconds or until smooth.
3. Pour into tall glasses and serve.

Peanut Butter Cup Shake

Serves: 2

Nutritional values per serving:

- Calories – 463
- Fat – 14 g
- Carbohydrate – 32 g
- Protein – 53 g

Ingredients:

- 2 cups skim milk
- 2 tablespoons peanut butter
- 2 scoops Creatine powder
- 2 large egg whites
- 5 scoops chocolate éclair protein powder
- ¼ cup hazelnut creamer

Method:

1. Add milk, peanut butter and creatine powder into a blender.
2. Blend for 30-40 seconds or until smooth.
3. Pour into tall glasses and serve.

Mass Gainer Shake

Serves: 2

Nutritional values per serving:

- Calories – 715
- Fat – 29 g
- Carbohydrate – 41 g
- Protein – 72 g

Ingredients:

- 1 cup ground almonds
- Stevia powder to taste
- 3 cups water
- 1 medium banana, peeled, sliced
- 4 scoops unflavored protein powder

Method:

1. Add ground almonds, stevia, water, and banana and protein powder into a blender.
2. Blend for 30-40 seconds or until smooth.
3. Pour into tall glasses and serve.

Creamy Peanut Butter Shake

Serves: 2

Nutritional values per serving:

- Calories – 461
- Fat – 16 g
- Carbohydrate – 46 g
- Protein – 37 g

Ingredients:

- 2 cups fat free milk
- 4 tablespoons peanut butter
- 2 scoops chocolate whey protein powder
- 2 medium bananas, peeled, sliced

Method:

1. Add milk, peanut butter, protein powder and bananas into a blender.
2. Blend for 30-40 seconds or until smooth.
3. Pour into tall glasses and serve with crushed ice.

Bring On Fitness

Chapter 5 - Breakfast Shakes

Oatmeal Shake

Serves: 2

Nutritional values per serving:

- Calories – 867
- Fat – 14 g
- Carbohydrate – 110 g
- Protein – 75 g

Ingredients:

- 2 scoops vanilla protein powder
- ¼ cup maple syrup
- 2 tablespoons chopped almonds
- 1 teaspoon ground cinnamon
- ½ cup raw oats
- 3 cups fat free milk

Method:

1. Add protein powder, oats, maple syrup, almonds, cinnamon and milk into a blender.
2. Blend for 30-40 seconds or until smooth.
3. Pour into tall glasses and serve with crushed ice.

Energy Blast Shake

Serves: 2

Nutritional values per serving:

- Calories – 1023
- Fat – 22 g
- Carbohydrate – 127 g
- Protein – 80 g

Ingredients:

- 4 scoops vanilla protein powder
- 1 cup raisins
- 2 tablespoons peanut butter
- 3 cups skim milk
- ¼ cup almonds, chopped
- 1 cup raw oats

Method:

1. Add protein powder, oats, peanut butter, almonds, raisins and milk into a blender.
2. Blend for 30-40 seconds or until smooth.
3. Pour into tall glasses and serve with crushed ice.

Banana Bread Shake

Serves: 2

Nutritional values per serving:

- Calories – 587
- Fat – 3 g
- Carbohydrate – 86 g
- Protein – 54 g

Ingredients:

- 4 cups water
- 1 cup cooked oatmeal
- 2 cups mashed bananas
- 4 scoops unflavored whey protein powder
- Powdered Stevia to taste
- 1 ½ cups bran flakes

Method:

1. Add all the ingredients into a blender.
2. Blend for 30-40 seconds or until smooth.
3. Pour into glasses and serve with crushed ice.

Fibrous Fruit

Serves: 2

Nutritional values per serving:

- Calories – 287
- Fat – 1.9 g
- Carbohydrate – 49.1 g
- Protein – 25.4 g

Ingredients:

- 2 cups milk or apple juice
- 2/3 tablespoon milk and egg protein powder
- 7-8 strawberries, chopped or 2/3 cup blueberries or 2/3 cup chopped peaches
- 1 cup wheat germ
- 1 banana, peeled, sliced, frozen
- 1 cup ice cubes

Method:

1. Add the fruits, milk, wheat germ, protein powder and ice into a blender.
2. Blend for 30-40 seconds or until smooth.
3. Pour into tall glasses and serve.

Breakfast Champion Shake

Serves: 2

Nutritional values per serving:

- Calories – 564
- Fat – 14 g
- Carbohydrate – 62 g
- Protein – 47 g

Ingredients:

- 2 cups skim milk
- 2 scoops vanilla protein powder
- 1 cup raw oats
- Ice cubes, as required
- 2 large egg whites
- 2 cups mixed berries of your choice
- ¼ cup almonds, chopped

Method:

1. Add the berries, milk, oats, whites, protein powder and ice into a blender.
2. Blend for 30-40 seconds or until smooth.
3. Pour into tall glasses and serve.

Egg-cellent Shake

Serves: 2

Nutritional values per serving:

- Calories – 578
- Fat – 13 g
- Carbohydrate – 40 g
- Protein – 46 g

Ingredients:

- 3 cups sugar free vanilla ice cream
- 6 whole eggs
- 4 scoops protein powder, unflavored

Method:

1. Add ice cream, eggs and protein powder into a blender.
2. Blend for 30-40 seconds or until smooth.
3. Pour into glasses and serve with crushed ice.

The Hulk Shake

Serves: 2

Nutritional values per serving:

- Calories – 148
- Fat – 1 g
- Carbohydrate – 9 g
- Protein – 25 g

Ingredients:

- 2 cups water
- 2 scoops vanilla protein powder
- 2 cups ice
- 1 tablespoon fat free pistachio instant pudding mix
- 2 teaspoons peppermint extract

Method:

1. Add ice, water, pudding mix, peppermint extract and protein powder into a blender.
2. Blend for 30-40 seconds or until smooth.
3. Pour into glasses and serve with crushed ice.

Chapter 6 - High Protein Shakes

Berry Good Shake

Serves: 2

Nutritional values per serving:

- Calories – 653
- Fat – 5 g
- Carbohydrate – 68 g
- Protein – 84 g

Ingredients:

- 30 blueberries
- 2 cups strawberries
- 4 cups nonfat milk
- 2 cups nonfat strawberry Greek yogurt
- 4 scoops protein powder, unflavored
- 2 cups ice

Method:

1. Add the berries, milk, yogurt, protein powder and ice into a blender.
2. Blend for 30-40 seconds or until smooth.
3. Pour into tall glasses and serve.

Sweet Strawberry

Serves: 2

Nutritional values per serving:

- Calories – 500
- Fat – 10.8 g
- Carbohydrate – 28.1 g
- Protein – 74.3 g

Ingredients:

- 2 cups water
- 4 tablespoons flaxseed oil
- 1 cup frozen strawberries
- 4 scoops vanilla protein powder
- 1 cup Greek yogurt

Method:

1. Add strawberries, water, flaxseed oil, protein powder and yogurt into a blender.
2. Blend for 30-40 seconds or until smooth.
3. Pour into tall glasses.
4. Serve with crushed ice.

Strawberry Energy Shake

Serves: 2

Nutritional values per serving:

- Calories – 876
- Fat – 4 g
- Carbohydrate – 131 g
- Protein – 79 g

Ingredients:

- 2 scoops protein powder, unflavored
- 20 whole strawberries, frozen
- Powdered Stevia to taste
- 3 cups water
- 1 teaspoon vanilla extract
- 2 cups ice

Method:

1. Add strawberries, water, vanilla, stevia, protein powder and ice into a blender.
2. Blend for 30-40 seconds or until smooth.
3. Pour into tall glasses and serve.

Caramel Hazelnut Shake

Serves: 2

Nutritional values per serving:

- Calories – 521
- Fat – 13 g
- Carbohydrate – 32 g
- Protein – 70 g

Ingredients:

- 4 scoops chocolate protein powder
- 3 cups fat free milk
- 2 tablespoons peanut butter
- ¼ cup whipped cream topping
- 2 cups ice
- ¼ cup nonfat Greek yogurt
- 2 tablespoons hazelnut creamer

Method:

1. Add protein powder, milk, peanut butter, whipped cream topping, ice, yogurt and hazelnut creamer into a blender.
2. Blend for 30-40 seconds or until smooth.
3. Pour into glasses and serve with crushed ice.

Double Berry Shake

Serves: 2

Nutritional values per serving:

- Calories – 861
- Fat – 1 g
- Carbohydrate – 73 g
- Protein – 140 g

Ingredients:

- 2 cups blueberries
- 2 cups strawberries
- 1 cup water
- 4 scoops protein powder, unflavored
- 2 cups ice

Method:

1. Add the berries, water, protein powder and ice into a blender.
2. Blend for 30-40 seconds or until smooth.
3. Pour into tall glasses and serve.

Tropical Pleasure Shake

Serves: 2

Nutritional values per serving:

- Calories – 531
- Fat – 6 g
- Carbohydrate – 50 g
- Protein – 71 g

Ingredients:

- 6 ounces pineapple juice
- 2 tablespoons heavy whipping cream
- 2 scoops protein powder, unflavored
- 2 cups ice cubes
- 2 cups water
- 1 teaspoon coconut extract
- 1 medium banana, peeled, sliced
- Stevia powder to taste

Method:

1. Add pineapple juice, cream, banana, coconut extract, Stevia, water, protein powder and ice into a blender.
2. Blend for 30-40 seconds or until smooth.
3. Pour into tall glasses and serve.

Super Peach Shake

Serves: 2

Nutritional values per serving:

- Calories – 825
- Fat – 17 g
- Carbohydrate – 93 g
- Protein – 76 g

Ingredients:

- 1 whole peach, deseeded, frozen
- 2 cups water
- 2 scoops protein powder, unflavored
- 2 tablespoons flaxseed oil
- 12 whole strawberries, frozen
- Stevia powder to taste

Method:

1. Add strawberries, peach, flaxseed oil, water, protein powder and stevia powder into a blender.
2. Blend for 30-40 seconds or until smooth.
3. Pour into tall glasses and serve.

Very High Protein Shake

Serves: 2

Nutritional values per serving:

- Calories – 971
- Fat – 5 g
- Carbohydrate – 74 g
- Protein – 158 g

Ingredients:

- 4 cups fat free cottage cheese
- 4 cups skim milk
- 1 cup vanilla nonfat Greek yogurt
- 6 scoops vanilla protein powder
- 1 cup strawberries, chopped
- Stevia powder to taste

Method:

1. Add strawberries, cottage cheese, milk, yogurt, protein powder and Stevia powder into a blender.
2. Blend for 30-40 seconds or until smooth.
3. Pour into tall glasses and serve with crushed ice.

Peanut Butter Gainer Shake

Serves: 2

Nutritional values per serving:

- Calories – 614
- Fat – 6 g
- Carbohydrate – 31 g
- Protein – 108 g

Ingredients:

- 6 scoops protein powder, unflavored
- 2 tablespoons peanut butter
- 2 cups ice
- 8 large egg whites
- 2 cups water

Method:

1. Add all the ingredients into a blender.
2. Blend for 30-40 seconds or until smooth.
3. Pour into glasses and serve with crushed ice.

Bring On Fitness

Conclusion

I want to thank you for again choosing this book. I hope you found some delicious recipes and that this book has been helpful in your endeavor to introduce healthy muscle-building shakes into your diet.

The book contains the best 50 muscle building shake recipes, which will help you strengthen your body from within by introducing fresh and healthy ingredients into your diet. To make it easier for you, we have ensured that all recipes are made using ingredients that are easily available at the local grocery store or farmers' market.

For best result, try to use fresh and organic produce. Also remember, muscle building is not only about what you eat, it is also a lot of hard work in the gym. Ensure you exercise consistently and drink ample water.

So what are you waiting for – let's get whirring that blender and get started!

Thank you, and remember to share how well these muscle building protein shake recipes work for you. You can do that by writing a review in your Amazon account under Your Orders.

Thank you,

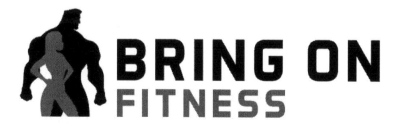

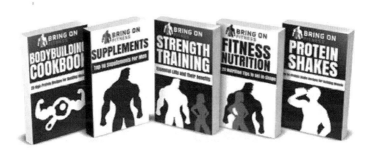

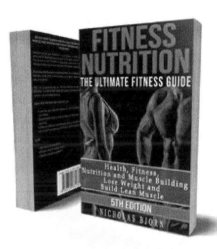

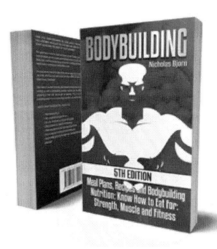

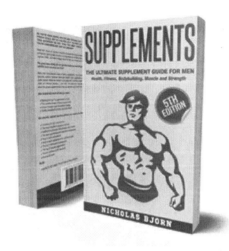

Printed in Great Britain
by Amazon

55672023R00043

To D

Thank you
for keeping
me alive
for So long

Ernie
Burns

Dedicated to my Mum and Dad,
my sister Veronica
and to Jackie, Elaine and Joseph
Thank you

The Bedlam Breakout

The guards of Bedlam
Were immersed in a fight
On the box
And were tight
So the locks
Weren't shut right
So, this night was the night
For one inmates flight

Pushing the cell doors
Gentle first then with force
That they swung was a source
Of utter surprise
Widening mad eyes
He suppressed his shocked cries
He could now break all his ties
With the disguise of the lies
Then rise
Off of new highs

Creep, creep
Little feet
Lull the world
Into a sleep
I will pass
Unto the street
Out a window
Down a sheet
Smother the sound
On the concrete
Into the shadow
Then retreat
While the world
Is fast asleep
Creep, creep, creep

So, out of Bedlam there was escape
But as, as ever, it came too late
They pulled it down
Built a new estate
That latter collapsed
Under its own weight

Bedlam was deemed too ugly to see
But look in a mirror
So are we

The Haircut
(Internally Yours)
(My Delilah)

It was to be another
Three weeks wait
To be inside your welcome
Inside your welcome face
To enjoy that easing easy grace
That mouths and tongues create
That would resonate
The gaping ache
Denial could not shake

That this was to be
Only
A haircut for a friend

You guided
The clippers' trace of shave
Skimmed my scalp
With its touch sigh
My hand impatient
Rose up
Under your dress
To rhyme
That clipping droned vibration
Replied with a thigh embrace
A tugging haste
Urged my hand to become enlaced

Your clit
Its spit
The sweet delicate split
Knits and unknits
Wet
And waiting

I'm internally yours
Surges roar and claw
Eternity
Whispered in licking kisses
As we never speak
Not that I want words
As I lay down on you
As you took me
My sweat
To skin
In, in
Internally yours

The Impotence of Being ...Earnest

Then you left
Me slightly broken
Smoking on the bed
Watching your silent sneak
To the proper berth
For your proper sleep
You took your leave
To dream on
In comfort

While In the hollow of my pillow
Still full of warm sighed breath
The haircut was complete

<u>Achieving failure</u>
<u>(A Self-help Guide</u>
<u>In One Easy Lesson)</u>

A small stake in this big town
That is all it takes
To make the changes necessary
Finally
    Forget
          The chances
Wasted
That had exploded
Into
A million catalogued shards

The improving pamphlet
Titled

Achieving failure

(All failures must be achieved)

Lesson one:

Cutting the air supply in order
To stimulate the need

Or:

How to be freed
From that evil side
That hides and hides
All snide wide eyed

Achieving failure

Are you are striving to be the saviour
To your own
Or searching for a saviour
To stop from feeling so alone

On Your Suicide

How could you say?
In that way that you did.
That was it
You had had enough
...Moreover, meant it.
I've missed the exit
At every attempt
But you just flew it
Like a girl possessed

They
must
have
 undressed
 you

Those who pressed you to the slab
Why weren't you naked in the bed anyway?
Who did you think was going to find you?
That was left for your mum to do.
I suppose you knew that

But the shock...
Just the type of selfish!

But, ok then...

...We will just leave it at that, then.

We have to
Because of your self obsessed
Unrepeatable act
That tiny step back
Into the black

Well... Bye.

You left me questions
That was your strange revenge
You purchased by dying
At your own hand
So boring and bland
You were right
I don't understand

Traditional Explosions
(November 5)

The to and fro of traditional explosions
Always raise surprised gasps
Of awe and
"Woo!"
Ever the spectacle rewards,
As sparkling flame soars

We cannot but delight
At how the ever 'ere evolves
How blue black night
Calls us
To its splendour
The turn of time revolves us
As a feather
In gusts of dusty wind

So it must be we pretend
That our minds' eyes
Did not know the start
What those whizzing booms
In miniature impart

Why would we "ooh!" and "ah!"
At this sight
If something deep inside us
Had not witnessed
The first explosion
That birthed light

<u>Bella</u>

She walks
Uncovering London
3.35am
The shooting summer melody of dawn
Cascades her slight frail dress
Flimsy floral shoes
Not much else to lose
...Apart from her way

Half along a street
She comes upon a door
Pauses to fix her full brown hair
The locks enswathe
Her plump rouged cheek
Pouting her full Italian lips
She frowns

It is quite apparent she has had too much
Perhaps she still craves a little more

She stretches up her hand
And shakes herself in tiny sways
That ripples
Folds of her sheer silk gown
After another pause
She reaches out
To rap upon the door

The Heave

The night traffic drones
A fibril web of juggernaut quakes
That shakes the brick
I shelter my worn bones
Unearthed beneath

Rays of stinging light
Streak the wet asphalt path
Outside shrieking that headache reassurance
That prayer of screaming
Declaring the hours
Where the day in shadow is illumed
By woken minds
Like mine
Marking the hid movement
Through the weave
On which persistence rests unevenly
Envisioning
No true essence
To our world
Only the fastening of souls
Founded in turmoil
And the expense expended
To maintain it all
That seems so far from our control
As if it were a gods' instruction.
But it leads alone to a self-destruction.

The Long Road

I do not want to leave,
Yet, we have to go,
This weight piles thick,
My muscles seem like stone,
I feel alone,
So ...just so,
And yes before you start,
I know,

Let's go, let us blow,
Flow upon the breezes that grow,
Up from the breathe of the below,
That holds firm the ragged sheath,
Covering the sharpness and the grief,
Of that sneaking coward thief,
Called time,
Who now I learns a friend of mine,
Let's celebrate our fates in wine,
Then take the long road home tonight,
The air is fresh and fine,
We are live and star aligned,
And the darkness is so kind,
As to make our visions bind,
Unravel then to wind,
Inside a blinded mind,
The one place we might yet find,
The   shape   of   hope   defined.

You Were Right All Along

You were right all along,
You cannot remember being wrong
There was no result but the one
That became the outcome
And you knew all along

No doubts, no confusion
No mistakes or delusions
No retributions
The conviction is strong
You knew all along

And now, that it is done
That the moment is gone
We have seen what went wrong
You tell everyone
You were right all along

But reversing foresight
Fashions a light
That burns much too bright
Until it, blinds like the night

So what you know and you knew
Seem no different to you
Does that make it true?
Had you really one clue?
Is your view not askew?

Are you sure, it was you?
Who was right all along?

The Train Again

I see you sitting there
Calling yourself me
That's the way it continues to proceed
We are peaceful people
So, we never really say
What it is we are feeling
We let slip...
...Another way

Failure Finally Achieved

I've done that
Been there
Overused the clichés
My failure, at long last
Can finally be achieved
I can then rest uneased

Reaching no target
Involved as much effort
If not more
With so many bores
To be bored
While I chore
A struggle for hard fought defeat
My goodness I do it so neatly
Completely on my own
The fallow fields I have sown
It overwhelms
I'm overblown
So when I take and bomb this test
In achieving failure
I will finally attain success.

Both Ways
(In search of the lost poet)

She chipped the cup
I smashed it
She bumped the car
I crashed it
She wrote the check
I cashed it
Sexism works both ways

Why You Hate Antiques

Acid taste of camphor
Wafts off the patina's grain glow
A table top of maple
Silk smooth
…And the cool touch
Worn by forgotten ways
Demands its price in praise

However, you see a cling of lost emotions
Only the dead have felt or understand
Strands of meaningless value
And I mean valued for a vault
Assaults you
As it should do for me

We must truly free ourselves
To live
We must have breath
To give our breath in effort
Then forget it, and forgive
Respect the spirit not the thing
Embrace the world
And bestow the gifts we bring

That must be why
You hate things that are old
We are too easily deceived
By the stories that they hold

How love is

The shined ebony plastic sack
Bloated in the kitchen corner
Filled brimming with microbes
Feeding on the dead rose
And the remains
Of the romantic meal

Their presence infects
Even our everyday
"I love you" s
Those are some how
Now twisted by an edge
Of resentment
For the moment's effort
The screwed up eyes
We have both avoided
It has haunted us all night
A war of duvet proportions
As we apportion
Less cover
For the other
Even if we smother ourselves

The bin no longer smells
It is a stench
That makes me wretch
And eventually wrench myself
From this restless rest
To take out the rubbish
That is…
Just…
So us…

Sitting Monkey

Sitting monkey on the wall
Sitting pretty
Standing tall
Tigers purr, triggers maul

Exhale the sigh,
Don't be denied

You are only weeping
For the tears you have cried

The air full flows
Then is tinted
A sensual hew
The ache
The joy
The angelic view
The world has loved us
Passing through
Feel its caress as it cradles you

Forgotten Dreams

Do they exist?
Do they?
Do they answer?
In hopeless un-mouthed
Pleas
Maybe we realise
In that fugue of inattentiveness
How to unify the race
Impose a reason on infinity
Or simply orgasm in repose
...Then sleep deeper

Could we in death connect to life in the same way?

The way we cling to our addictions
Grasp at our religions
Try to disavow our connection
To the flesh we have become

How can the fragrance of existence
Become so distant

That we must awake
Shape light and forget
The unremembered dreams
Our oblivious minds have met

The Librarian Revolution

She needed the radiators bleeding
So, I had to find out what to do
In a "how to" book
I thought the library worth a look

But she was already there
Giving me that squinty stare
Used to make me feel abused
And she tapped her foot
Inside her pointy
Dust touched shoe
Folded her arms
Then told me
What I could do...

She said

"You think so thinly
You think I am meant to act so primly
But I do not shush!
There is no hush
Except the one inside your mind
The book that you need to find
...Is titled

"Choose Sight Do Not Be Blind"

...But are you listening?
You're dumbly pointing at the Dewy number 807.3
This is not "D I Y"
But in fact "Art Philosophy"
A mistake
That is made so frequently
It's like a spike being driven in me

But I have grace and ease
In my heart I long for peace
Give me poetry please

I have to have these sympathies
No matter how tattered they're meant
It's just that it's time that you went"

...Then the library closed shut
Those impressive doors
With a thud
Of prestigious philanthropy
Embodied in the fact
The dogma of the dead

Was still connected to the thread
We tread along
As we go on
So, I went on
Left her Behind
And her mind
And her kind

Too Much Money Not Enough Grace

Surrounded and bound by Savil Row stitches
I cannot suppress an urge
To pick at their insecure twitches
As we pass a pub in Temple
Called

"The Witness Box"

Their rich laughter sounds thin
Over their gin cocktails
That defines their disciplines' exploitation
The polite terror they inflict
Accompanied by the spittle spit
That expresses their passions
As it hits us in the eyes
Those snorts rise
And their performance turns into palaver
They get in a "lather"
While consuming consolation

"This is the life, nice kids, nice wife,
Nice whiff of the slice of cake"

The little more they deserve and take

A greed that turns hatefully
Away from the victims in its wake

"Oh, It's all right I can step on you,
I am wearing an Italian designer shoe"

Barley Juice and the Broken Break

There was a busy man
Outside a public house
Beer gardening
With a whiskey

"This is the life." He surmised

Not knowing any better
Raised his glass
To make his whistle wetter
Enjoyed the satisfied sigh
Exhaled with a tide of relaxation
As he searched for...
A deeper reclined position
In this easing seat

The sweat, which had seeped
From his brow
A dim unbelievable memory
That seemed as if almost
A snippet of a documentary
Something off TV
He had watched but had not seen

Then a ring of polyphonic tone
Heralded an urgent call from home
So, he drove back
Into the back of a eighteen wheeler
The police report did not highlight
Any distinct relaxed demeanour

Black Holes Beings

We are singular
Folds in space
Uniquely spaced
Within ourselves
The place of names
We share and yet…
Wholly contain alone
In our event horizon home

Smoking (adjective) Kills (noun)

Flows of particulate vapour
Breaking gravity's press
Streams up from the gash
Smashed into the head
Of the fallen crumpled victim
On the harsh, hard pave
Not porous enough to absorb
The pooling black red
Seeping from the scar

In the cold
The steaming hole
All wrong and beyond
Help or expectation
The thoughts spilling
To the ground
With the echo of the cracking
Smacking
Splashing
Pop
The dizzy realisation that
Everything will stop
Like the final spasm spins of a faltered
Spinning top

Fixated on the fight to catch the light
In the prism of the night
Next to his blearing eyes
From pocket spills
Printed on a tobacco product packet
Reads the legend…
"Smoking Kills"

Mystic Shit Mandala

Your contacts
Left in a teacup
By the bedside
Had stained a tannin brown
The cup was not clean
So the lenses opaqueness
Irritated vision
They had swelled slightly
Causing a haze of stinging sight
You did not right it
In the night
As you had meant and said you would

But you had had another swig instead
It went, of course, straight to your head
Still you sang
"Maybe"
With a smile
"I can go another mile"
Then the widdershins ensued
You envisioned
In blindness
The reasons for the spell
Lucid as blood
How it shocks us
When it is out of place
You paled

You had seen the future
It had touched you
With its absolute illusion
That it has not already passed

Brown ruby tinted now
The scorch of eating life
Eating at your eyes

I saw pictured
In your pleading scream
An outside to the dream
The world was captured in your mouth
Explaining all
In a kitsch allegory
You were the mandala
Containing everything within

Edges Aspirations

Edges maintain their dreary drudge
Attending to their eternal job
Defining what is and what is not
Performing radical surgery
On objects in our presence

Edges can not help this
They serve

Yet, do they yearn to smudge the order they endure?
Play like words do
Turn chairs into human legs
Then brake them
On concrete deep shag pile carpets
Covering the chests of giant bonobos' fleas
Feasting on skin scales left as treats
Howling to be discovered as they hide

But edges only dream,
Though they have no time for dreams
They carry on
Separating atoms
And stop us from reading minds
I am grateful
Thank you edges
For your diligence

Untitled
(Unblossoming)

I see etches in
my palm
Retracing growth
 and birth
Past all confines
Into the other death

              ...Before life

In this blindness
These spirit eyes
Witness an abyss
Stealing even words

           ...Taking even this

Untitled
(You as water)

Your hair once flowed black rivers
Into the shores of my hands
But drained grey suds
In ebbing

As
My hands parted

Lips tightened

My hands are a bone dry
Desert
Eroding memories
In hot storms

Hungry Woman

The meal congealing
Solidly
In front of her
On the draped table
A marinated duck sucked dry
Of nourishment as it hung
Long before it hit a plate
She sips rose wine
With contemplative glances
To other dinners
Involved in their other parties

Small puddles of plum sauce
Firming on the vitreous porcelain
Reflect her considered
Carefree smiles
Toward the head waiter
Who lets her eat here
And will let her pay
With the anecdotes of émigrés
From migrated kitchens

"No" She laughs, it is her craft
How she captures her career
Licking her lip of salt
She stalls, still hungry
Still she cannot eat another bite

The six strips of tepid meat
Delicious despite the lateness
Of the early morning night
Rich and as moreish
As the delicacies
She will not eat

Her stories long to loll of her tongue
Her dark skin glistens in the candle glare
The scars less apparent
The truth is a knife of cold hard steel
Spins and alights on watchers
And their stares toward her connect
Calls them over
As they invite themselves to spare chairs
Where they seat instead of leaving for the street
Where they should have been

The aimless talk begins
Ritual transactions
As elaborate

As instinctive
As they are ancient
She feeds to them from fingers
The callused unforgiving edge
That had made her bed
In the old rich mans house
And how the baby boy son is not a man
Because he resents
This she all presents
In exchange for the tales telling
And what she can get
To make the hunger less

Pizza Perfect Tense

Carrying in his undersized hands
A sizeable eighteen inch box
Horizontal flat as not to disrupt
The toppings spilling from the crust
A hunger with a name and personality
Hangs inside his hung over head
That moved up from his guts
To perform a take over bid
Overriding cognition
A contrite admission
...That, though slowly poisoning himself
He does not want to die
Death is not his thing

The impotence of being ...Earnest

The pizza squirms greasily
Underneath its cardboard sheathe
A breaded cheesy wreathe
He will lay his dreams beneath
Sleep on as a pillow
Though it is hacked
With the marks of teeth

World

We thought we were being brought together
We were, in fact being driven apart
Torn asunder
Little wonder

We could have been resting in each others arms
I let my stupid pride have sway
Let you recede further than I should
Until I could not reach out

I have been convinced
My touch is poison
It has never done me any good

You... you have the world
At your finger tips
All I ever wanted was to give
And so I must give
Let love in
And simply live...
Real

It...Is...NOT...real
It must be said
Repeated
This is not real
As the knife goes in
Into the
Seams on reams of paper
Thin forearm skin
Bleeds on black and white
Bleeds on
In libraries and files

This is real
Not understood

Real
Not filled with meaning

And you learn eventually
You have to say to yourself
keep on
Keep on saying
This is NOT real

Silent God

Hey God!
Why so coy?
Why the big silence that, you employ?
Is it?
That your mysterious ways
Are the crazy paves to some form of enlightenment?
Or after the first seven days
Did you feel an entitlement to an early retirement?

But why remain silent?

Then watch our suffering
Safe and afar
Beneath your celestial covering

When there are things we need to know
Questions that are worrying us

Like:

Would Jesus have done the same?
If he really knew the pain
That would follow in his name

Dear God, please explain?
It should be simple and so plain...
...Again, you just refrain
It seems it is not worth saying
That you are only playing

Still, it is not too long a wait
To see
Though by then it is too damn late
To alleviate the hate
That one word would obviate

So if we are here for your amusement
My disgust will cause no bemusement
But if you are love then you will forgive
My sceptic's doubt and let me live

Omnipotence should know why I persist
Asking why is Heaven dumb
If it really does exist?

We Let Them

The seasons change
We let them
The seas churn
We let them
The skies thin
We let them
The earths rip
We let them
The stars hum

We believe that we allow
The movements of the universe
If not us our image or its curse

The politicians lie
We let them
The rich deny their greed
We let them
The bullies crush
We let them

The dictators figurehead
This Medusa ship of fools
That employs death to float
We let it
Participate in it
Either blind or weary eyed
Or just trapped so deep inside
This selfish murder ride

We let it
Allow that

Refute that this is truth
Think the dreams a sweeter fruit

Me Versus Me

"Fight!"
I shouted
To encourage the combatants
Complacent, as I was, to be
Spectator not contender
The unexpected punch in my face
Caused a rip in my cheek
The skin beneath the eye
Is very, very weak
it caused blood to release
Like shaken fizzy pop but thicker
I fell collapsing to the floor
Where I got a kicking off a kicker
It cracked my skull and atrophied my ticker

So, I only whisper fight now
Even if I am watching on T.V
But still I want to witness
Still I have got to see

What Poets Do

It is what the poets do
Mumble in there solitary rooms
Of how the echo booms
Against their Skulls

They remove their minds away
To some other
Spiritual place
Between the sight and gaze
Then attempt to leave some trace
In the emptiness of space
That surrounds and grounds us

A Purpose of Dreams

There are two dreams that circle night
Born in blindness or borne on light

They feed on us, we feed on them
They mirror fire and icy gem

The fleeting span of a glints glean
That hits an eye but still's unseen

The same power, as an embrace
Those connections that touches trace

They faintly brush our solid dust
We grasp their shades they crumble rust

A faded flash a silenced shout
The memory that fills with doubt

How dreamt attempts leave so exposed
The eye left open, the eye left closed

<u>It was in your Name</u>

"So, what?"
You sighed
Emerging from the dark green light
Dappling through the trees
You spoke as if what you had faked
For so long
Was finally true
At last you could ignite that furious song
To serenade
My failing
Zero superhero ego...
Ergo...

But you were wrong
The blood had splattered us all
You would find our names
There
On the monument to survivors
That would or could not be built
Depicting the violence
That goes unexplained

It was beginning to get late

"Oh?" You choked "So "you" know?"
"Whatever." I said
But I meant
"Never mind."
"You should be seeing, really seeing."
"Not that peek-a-boo peeping."
"That you pursue."
"Its touched us too."
"Because we all call ourselves me."
"So it was me,
See, me!
And that includes you"

It was in our name
With no way
For us to exclude the pain
Discount ourselves excused
From any of the blame

It is the simple price we pay
To use the numbers on the money
Or the numbers of the day

The Start of Another
Nine And A Half Years

You long for sleep
So, I'll go
With no tears
I've waited months
I've waited years
And my fears of waiting
Are long gone
So I do not mind
And will move on

Temperance
(How Everything Engulfs)

Her indifference worn
As if it were make up
She wears her thoughts
As if they are made up
A pretend belief
A grief as armour she adopts to be adored
Pouring water
From one vessel to another
Mimicking
The temperance tarot card
A futile action
Attracts attention
Greater than intention's works demand
And slanders are compliments to her
Confusion her vital element
And all is spent on vanity
Or letting go
Of pointless vanity

Do not pretend the surface
Is not all there has to be
You lie and lie
But you are not free

To see

What is hidden here beyond

How the turn of life goes on

Alien Attitudes

I lived the future
It wasn't much
Not so different
It was still a wasteland

I broke the surface
With the can tab's psst
The real thing melted
In a soda pop
As the spacemen call it

But nothing came of it

This time machine is kaput now
It keeps me in the same moment
Just microseconds away from the beautiful aliens
I want to introduce them to my possible present

So, I bought the future
It wasn't much
Only cost half a lifetime

And my central core

The mist has not dispersed on this dawn
Must be the radiation

So, do you want to know the future?
No, I didn't think so....

Personally I wouldn't change a thing
Apart from the time, circumstance and location

The Bus of Tourettes

Facing the frets of people
Not letting his gibbering
Get to them
He carries on
His carry on
He cannot help how it
SPURTS out
Those MAD shouts

An echo
Like the tracks
Of a train
Crissing
Crossing
And sparking his brain
Begging for order
For that squandered thirty-four years
The taxing arrears
Of the loss of the peace
That expelling the mess
May still achieve
The mess he sees around him
Outside of his head
That is not madness
That is real
Abuse
I am using as fuel
For my own inane babble
An hysteria to steal
With tiny finger twitches
That might reduce them
A peg or two
The bitches
That stitched
My rage and fury together
And I now wear
As I wear away

"You are lucky mate!"

No one will touch you

That dementia
Cannot confront
Only affront
And confuse
We all have
Too much to lose

Long Day

I have counted the seconds today
Attempting to relieve the doubt
That had wormed sleekly
Into my mind
That I had been lied to about time

It began in my youth
In an incident
When I had noticed
That I had aged faster than I should
But I had put it down
To being run down
By a runaway bus
That had careered
Along the high street
Taking out shop fronts
And litter bins
The driver laughing
As it tumbled

So I counted my years of torment
Mouthed the seconds
In and out
And now I have found
The shocking truth
There were forty four more
Than the eighty six thousand four hundred
That there should have been
Forty four seconds
Unaccounted for in the myths
That tooled the day
That I have wasted away
Counting

The Racket Rule

Corrupt and cruel
The racket rule
Turns us into fools
Who simply drool
Fixed on the jewels
We use to fuel
The rotten rule

We are the tools
The greedy mules
That fill the pools

We school ourselves
In this cool induction
Smothering each other
In the rank corruption

Then turn to dust
And turn to drink
And turn the bloody wheel

Faceless
Avoiding any stare
Fearing what we may see in there
In a gaze
We would face
All the errors
Of our malign ways
The perfect denial to our shame
A banal and blameless blame

That the world is flat
The universe square

And in all that
No life can be found there
And a beating heart
Is a secret pain to bare
Until the lies
Are all that we share
Or care for

Over Poetry Death Has No sway
(Coroly to Ovid)

Over poetry death has no sway
The rhythm and the rhyme
Never wholly fade
It lives on past our finite lives
In the space our hearts inlay
However time erodes its mark
It can always live again

Still, poetry has no sway over death
Its meter must be conveyed
Upon a wet and living breath
It endures eternity
Yet the certainty, is clear
The poem is eternal
The poet 's not I fear

Continuity

She... noticed...continuity...
Had stopped...working...
That reality ...was somehow
...Broken
She knew that...
That man had worn his parting
On the other side...
When he sat down
But now...
It had clearly...
Changed position...
...It was a fact
Not a mere deluded supposition

...And the low cut dress
She had splurged out on
...On her card
Did add pounds...around her hips
Contrary to what she had been told
...And Alan had been laughing
Seconds before the laughter broke
...Revelations to provoke emotion
That salted cheeks with silver streaks
...As she reached out for...
The chair
That ...had been there
She landed hard below her feet

Then the rhythm skipped a...
Skipped a...
...Skipped a beat

Back at home with the hangover
She no longer remembers as her own
The theory and the facts don't meet

Elvis and Jesus in Vegas
(Any Similarity between Persons Living or Dead is Purely
Coincidental)

Elvis and Jesus
In a casino bar in Vegas
Popping fifties into the waitresses' g-strings
Drinking High-balls, Zombies
And "Long Island Iced Teas"
Talking about paradise puffing on stogies
Elvis had a connoisseur's taste for the "crazies"

They were just back from the Black Jack table
Elvis had kept his cool but Jesus was unable
He had lost because he had said "stick."
Instead of "hit me." and was busted stony

"All superstars gotta get their kicks
It is important for their equilibrium"
Elvis explained
Like he wasn't busting for a fix"
And why should they deny us this
One quick stop off at a snow white bliss

By now it was passed time, to move their itchy feet
Take in the show, or out to the street
Reap the rewards of the adulation
Elvis having been subject to the presses' speculation
That he and Jesus were more than just friends
So it all turned into a vilification and so crucified again
They shuffled off home to the top floor
The room decorated with diamonds
Even though Jesus had spent his allowance
What he was allotted,
"By god!"
And as he worriedly totted up the bill in his head
Elvis smiled sweetly, this is what he said

"I have more money than sense
I'll cover you Jesus
But you gotta repent"

Jesus shrugged saying
"What can I say?"
"This is the true heaven"

As cars collided
Outside the Penthouse
Bursts of bubble bullets
From automatic repeaters
Exchanged details

That filled mortician's reports
Weather forecasts
Police forensic reports
With this cold harsh fact

Jesus had learnt tact
But Elvis was fat

Piccadilly

I listen to the bawling boom
That covers something
That can't be shown
That is not for show
Especially for you

The impotence of being ...Earnest

The devil'd like to shake your hand
As if you shook the world
Well you wished you had
In his felt hat do you feel engulfed

Smothered by a strange talent
To stick your head into a vice
And the eternal light
That never goes out
Soon will be snuffed

But it is essentially stupid
Like blaming your bane on Cupid's bad memory
As you flew bye he forgot to fly an arrow
Through your heart

So, Piccadilly
Who's a whore now?

She is a Movie Today

She said she felt like a movie today
I said that "Star Wars" would be appropriate
Because she's always saying
She looks like "Jabba the Hut"

But I did not mean it to cut
As much

She tilted her head and made wrinkles
Round her eyes
And still I was surprised
By how angry she was
At the fact
That I had said something stupid
…Again

"Well, we'll go out…
…To a film
Watch what you want"

But it did not help
She thought that
I should
Understand
If anyone could
That she had meant
Something different than that…
Meant that she wanted out

"Like in the pictures
They always want out
And then the titles
And the tears
Fade in the light
Because sometimes
You go in the day
But mostly at night
No matter
In the end it always is bright"

But I only smiled
Pretending that I did see it the same
Like the illusions of patterns
Reflecting off silver are seen in the eye
But message distinctly
In each individuals mind

So she became her movie
In the end
A romantic comic tragedy
The sort popular nowadays
But the type I don't attend

Optimal Pessimism

You misheard
I said opportunist
Not optimist
You do not deserve this
But I'm showing your mistake
For the FUTURE
So, you KNOW
I know NOW
How much greed you will allow
And the stuff you are willing to break

Untitled
(On The Way toward Catford)

Part ONE

Cleopatra knew pain as all the eyes
That dried the dessert with their gaze stared her way
A desiccating observance

As the azure fraying silk
That barely covered what she desired
To be desired
Burnt
She learnt true cruelty
Her fidelity fading in the shouts

Thin flesh a gate to the fire
Screeched oils in response
Cried the slain phantom moan
Lovers pretend away
She would live fevered
In her centre and the sun
Forever

Part TWO

Her venom has insight
It knows the path of hearts
It takes on journeys
Tears apart the skies
Then the skies lose themselves

The spirits talk cloud
Talk mirror words
Take on form
Are Ignored
Or are called angels

She touches the empty fireplace
With the love she has explained
Within philosophies
Ordered in tranquillity
She faces the stark stack of the darkness
We only knew before we had eyes
Still she is surprised
How her body tries
To cling to explanations
That cannot save her

I reach out

Words Goodbye

As your friends
Condense into word
What we will miss about you
In the way that we have to do

It shows how hollow words are
How faint their touch
How inadequate a shroud they weave
How they miss you too

We'll say

"You loved life"

But not
Why you could not live it

We'll say

"You where the soul"

But not
Why we cannot forgive

That you will not be there
With those immaculate flaws
That begged applause
From the gods
Your grace with the odds
Riled against you
The care you took
To always, look beyond both ways
The crazy laughing days
Even the irritating gazes straight through
For real
And your beautiful playing
With the diamonds that fell at your feet
All incomplete

Words can only trace the dance
That you were so devoted to
It is why they seem so empty
They can't make your death less true

(Dedicated to Wendy)

Funny Bone

There is a funny peculiar bone
That has grown inside his brain
Into the shape of a question mark
It is as sharp and jagged
As the tooth of a shark
It cuts and strips and in the dark
It shines inside his mind

Bigger and bigger now
It is as big as his big ideas
Feeds on his thoughts for sustenance
And spears
All expectation
Expecting something
In return

Apart from a burning
It only tickles as it shreds
It talks bullshit and it begs
An independent life
A kid to fuck up
And a wife
To knock up too
And a god to lick its shoe
It plans to enlarge
And break the skull
In barrage of common sense
All cliché and so dull
He has kept it under drapes
But eventually when it escapes
Like the birth of Zeus' last mistake
A war will then ensue
One that will affect us too
An apocalyptic hullabaloo
Of the peculiar funny bone coup

And so...
We will drive
Through tears of pig blood rain
Along roads
Lined with victims
That we will call progress
Hurting and hating
That, that we do not understand,
But are desperate to possess
We will bow to the bone
In an orgy of excess

Accident

Shores wear
Slowly sometimes
Sometimes all as one
Falling like children tumble
But taking houses into rivers
Relative distance cannot be altered
The space between objects is constant
Only time changes

The grey lozenge legs hoisting road above water
Lasted one thousand seconds before exploding
Remembering themselves again as powder
Delicate lattice ripples of undertow
In mud
All that is left for the land
As recall
Of the surge
Until the next
Embrace

You Hit Harder at Night

Like the sparking carriages
Of night trains
Distancing themselves
Or nearing junctions
Are louder without light
In the dark
You fight harder
You hit harder at night
And the screams
Of the reversing trains
Mirror the dreams
That disturbs the kids
Is it that we want to live more?
When the sun is gone from our sight
Is that why
You hit harder a night?

The impotence of being ...Earnest

<u>Good Intention Boulevard</u>

You trip
        On a cracked pavement slab
Cut your knee
        So it will require stitching
You shrug
        And disappear
In an apologetic escapology
        A Hudiniesque escape
        Like you ate shadows
                To become shadow

Still blood trails will lead the way
        Blood tells on the street
        In the dark

I follow
        To an alley
                Good Intention Boulevard
        The home of a friend of a friend
A bust urban build up
        Rubbish and junked belongings
                To wade through to get to you
                        And your, by now, ink stare

The impotence of being ...Earnest

And I'll hold you
        But then let go
Not knowing
        How to grasp tighter

                Though I intended to

Wasn't it intentions
        That sent it all to hell

                So it is just as well, then

Untitled
(Because You Prefer No Title)

"Like rainbows then"
You laughed
"We will be rainbows."
And ran
As illusive
Unreal
And aloof

Dancing down the street
Like us
Beyond touch
And traffic
I could be light again
Feeling the energy freeing
From the shock of you
That even on a dark dry night
Rainbows can do as they like
They just pass sooner from our sight

My Muse Moved On

I have a phone number
It repeats in my slumber
I can remember it
But...
That's just bullshit
Because if I called HER!
No one would answer
She would not be THERE
And if she was
She would pretend
Thinking our non-relationship should end

Branding me

"Liar, liar
Brain on fire
Put the rest
Upon the pyre"

...And I would agree with her

So eventually, one day
I say
"Enough"
Time to slay
The monsters of cock
Who want me to stop
Full stop
All the trite slop
I use as my crop
And phone
To commune
With my muse

But she'd moved on

I don't hate Humans
(I don't think they are merely scum
I just detest the people they become)

I saw a white chalk legend
In a victim's angry scrawl
A pavement bulletin
Declaring to the world

"ALL HUMANS ARE SCUM"

I thought that's not right at all
It should say

"ALL HUMANS ARE CUM"

So I wrote that on a wall

The Door to Deceptions

Fluid oils off aged and clotted brilliant gloss
Chokes acidly tightening my throat
As the lid of the paint pot flips off
Inhaled it streams
Through my welling eyes in reflex
And spills
Upon the bristle of the sodden carpet
Making the mites all white
If they could seen with microscopic sight
And then they'll die

The bathroom door caked
In years neglect
Still needs cutting in
But will open upon a new future
Of productive hygiene
And rewarding ablutions
Encouragingly preaching
Life is to be embraced
As an end in itself
And not as a race

But sticky, stinking,
Impure one coat paint
That is decayed
Drips
Running down scarring
Like the veins in a addicts arm
As they fade and collapse

I am only scrapping the surface
Of all the disappointments, I will know
So in this substandard whitewash I will bathe
Smothered in its clutch I will be replaced
Nothing wasted, as I am suffocated
A seal to my disgrace

But the paint knows it is all lies
In the end, not the door but it's finish
That is the one more wise

Bus stop!

"Bus! Stop! Now!"
I sounded the bell
I shouted out…
…STOP!

The impotence of being ...Earnest

It is not the right place
But I will face that
And the consequence
Of my decision
The aggressive nature of my position
I'll kick up an exhibition
And embarrass everyone round me
Including… let's see
There is only me

And as I leave the bus
At the wrong alighting point
My overwrought screams
Are stinking like a joint
Burning pock mark holes
In the upholstery
And in the gantry
Flames lick
Next to a crack whore
Picking up scabs
Off the oil soaked floor
All zombie life is here
But I've seen it all before,
Before

Off the broken bus shattered I fall
Past the hissing stuttering
Slow to open door
I'm thinking
Why do I now have to walk?

When your mouth is shut
You should not talk

Solo Sunday

Wasted another look down
Through a blind of dust
And water stains
Onto the emptied
Seven a.m.
Sunday streets
Missing
The resting milk floats
Now souring
In the depot
Next to the terminus
The cricket ground of Edmonton
Where graffiti proclaims

"Crossroads are for the dead"

I turn back into a room
That turns more into me
The longer I look
Almost as vacant

Last days are always lonely
In a good way sometimes
Silvering to mirror
Not splinter

Still I cannot stop tending
The green shoots of the lie
Growing in the casual glance window box
I have built beneath the sill
…That someone
Will appear out there and care

The edit said It

They did not need to say it
Because the Edit said it

We did not to hear it
We'd been already fed it

The spiritual images
Of cleaner dishes

Promises of freedom
To get us in a fizz

That property portfolio
Did the vital bus-i-ness

Moves like a swan
But peek beneath the dress

You would never ever guess
It's a frantic business
That leaves a bloody mess

Cara's Poem

Desperate on a dizzy edge
Oblivion is all you beg
You ignore the bids
For a warmth touched bed
A stranger who will make room
For shame to be fed

Gagging on the casual abuses
He uses to express irrepressible want
All he wished christened in a sweat filled font

Clammily resisting his misdemeanours
He believes she'll go the way of all dreamers

"It did not kill us
We were only left
A little less alive
Inside
But we still survived
It was inside we died"

There may be no fabled knight
Charging in a light
That would banish 'ever night
She will need
More than religion
Or reason
To win her hard fought fight
To keep her eyes as bright

<u>Money is The Drug</u>
<u>Even its Dealers Abuse</u>

As is it is rolled
And it is folded
It gets dirty
Begins to smell
Of sweat, grease
And a species
Of bacteria
That eats
That micron thin layer of dust
That encrusts its worth

And in this we trust

Spiral Fly

Fly spiral fly
Land and lie low
Keep a wafer profile
Out of sight
Viral invisible
Indivisible from air
Quench your thirst and hunger
Then buzz a buzzing scoff
At us
Travelling in such a different
Direction
Detecting nothing of what you detect
With your compound eye

So, spiral fly
Go on and fly

Language is a Disease

Language
Before life
Spanned the universe
Spun spiralled order
Inertia
Weight and heat together
Eating void, exhaling time
An effort to form a prayer
To match the pulse throb oscillation
Existing before existence

Newly ripped from sleep
Alone grown weaker and sickened
Language burned to find words
To cure itself
Began tainting
The debris crystals
Of air rock and water
Floating
Folding their tangles
To express mass
Infected flesh dialects
To treat its unique disease
But lost all recollection
Of what it had been once
And never healed

Why Green Triangles
Started the Revolution From
Quality Street Boxes

The green triangles detested the rest
On the map
Thought them gaudy, plebeian
And so common
That they would say
"...As muck"
And be actually proud…

The green triangles didn't think the same way
They had different design aspirations
They saw
The "Ikea" like future
And prepared
While they waited for it to come

Still, living with those vulgar purples, pinks and gold toffees
Provided enough Excuse for them to protest
By shocking fillings on occasion
In the name
Of the future furniture revolution

Human Lab Rats

Rats and humans are alike
They both spike their hair with product or by-products
And they both eat wires and wireless technology
With no apologies, and they both cow tow
To the latest dictator the king felator
Who, licks privates in public
And they both wear the coarse uniform
Of natural selection putting everything in their station
Predator or prey, black or white, straight or gay

In a lay by, by the A604
She sips back a coke
It hits the back of her throat
And she feels disappointed
She wanted more;
More length,
More foreplay
More love,
More vodka in her cup
Her complexion, now pinker than red
She recites in her head
"I'm going to leave you soon"
And watches as he sparks a cigarette sated
Scratching his balls because he thinks
"That the right thing to do after sex"
She does not let him detect
That it is "so" nearly over
She keeps it together
And faintly remembers the time before
She no longer thought it was a pervy thing
Shaving herself, shaving him

Meanwhile in a university town
Animal activists free the experiments
And berate the terrible crime the pied piper committed
Leading rats to a river

"And if he'd been half decent
He'd have bought them a dinner first"

Or a snack, a crumb goes a long way
In a rat's estimation
That is what leaves them open to such exploitation
But come the revolution
When all confusion evaporates
The rats will put their tormentors in a maze
And instead of cheese
There will be money in the traps
And instead of disease, they'll spread love

The impotence of being ...Earnest

He drives her back to her parent's house
"How things are" plays on the radio
A song she finds to be such a coincidence
It had to be planned by the hands of the rats
Not the man

Mind over...
Doesn't matter

"Ten pennies for a miracle?
No?
Two then?
Less then?
...free?"

The more fantastic the illusion contrives to appear
The more convinced, the audience will be that it is real
That the sliced woman did resurrect
From fatal wounds
And flew above their heads
And became an angel

The initial reports declared
That she (Princess Diana)
Had only injured her legs
And may recover...
Comments that were latter forgotten
In the conflagration of speculations and ill formed opinions
Proffered by the pundits, required
By the shock of it all

A grandmother had also died that night
In a house fire
Caused by a fault in a plugged in television set
Luckily, the flames were controlled
Before spreading to rest in the terrace
She was asphyxiated.

Skip to two years later
The eve of a new millennium unable to live up the gravitas of
its name
In a crack house in Edmonton, north London
Nearly dead Tony Davis
Made a teary resolution to change his ways
Get his shit together, pack in the junk and...
"Sort it owtah!"
He did
But it only lasted seconds
Before he found out
He was... if "not weak", then "not strong"

He got back home two days later
Smelling of trouble
To find his wife leaving with the kids and the car
As he got to the gate
They drove passed his hurt and confusion
While neighbours and on lookers gawked laughing

He felt like his favourite trick
Those rings that look eternally linked
But come apart with no effort from the magician
And he laughed too

The fake charity she now works for sells donated second
hand clothes
To third world retailers who indirectly harm the micro-
economics of corrupt African oligarchs with international
interests
She is saving to pay to remove the tattoo of his name from
her arm
And a console or a hand held for the kids

The Dream of Dreamers

The dream of dreamers dreaming dreams
All called me
Uniquely

Asleep in velvet stars
Upon a crust of dust
Measuring a spark length light
Comprised of an eternal edge
Contained between the fine line
Of what is meant
And what is said

The True Eternals
(Rhyming time and time and time and time again)

There are few eternal truths
To the universe
Everything changes
In the changes in time
Dissolves, realigns
Redefines itself in time
Is minutely refined
Even truth changes
In time
Even justice
Language
But not rhyme
Poetry is eternal and...
Hope also
They both live on longer than Time

One Temple Said to the Other

One temple said to the other

"I am greater. I have the moon on my side"

The other replied

"I have darkness on my side"

One temple said to the other the other

"My King is bigger"

The other replied

"I have the clouds on my side"

The other replied

"But I have love on my side"

Then the temples fell
And I walked on into the night.

If Drugs are the Answer?
(What is the question?)

If drugs are the answer...
...What was the question...again?

Oh!
Am I happy?
Whatever
Are you?

There you are cutting your toes
To spite your nose
In spite of the benign tumour
That grows

Then dawn drawn across skies of tiles
And chimney stacks
Makes us cry ...laughter
As life returns
After the moon tricks of the lunatics
And their cold humours
That still play dances
On our closed eyes

Heavy Shit Got to Quit(
Got to Quit This heavy Shit)

I'm gonna give it up
I'm gonna recover
...After another
"Whose it gonna bother brother"
I don't feel right
I feel light
Like I'm floating
To that black hole exit
Hovering my head
Yet, I'm not dead
Only, badly led astray...

Heavy shit, gotta quit

Did you ask me...?
I did not answer
I did not care to
Interrupt the moment with remark
Break the still air with the yell
I would have had to let erupt
So I remained restrained

But heavy shit I'm gonna quit

Evil and good fight
Like the sperm and egg
A small scale tragedy
Played out everyday
Then dribbled down her leg
Entertained by some exotic freak
No mouth, only teeth
That chew the flesh to speak
Another unjust sleeper
Cannot break the sleep and sleeps
Like a shotgun kissed his flesh with beads...

Heavy SHIT! Time to quit

Sucking in the anger, I regret
The short sharp trap of breath
That became the nature of her grace
The name she put to faith
The step within the pace
The furrows she pained to trace
Across her brow
And then erase
But she can find no ease to smooth
The crease of frown

That carries sympathy for my disease
She can only mind to freeze
To etch that tattoo,
Of that pierced heart
That scar
The monument inside her breast

...heavy shit.... i... am really... going to quit

Conformed into an angle of divine desperation
Torn, exposed, tattered
And oh so titillating
Taking in roughly moulded exhalations
To the flesh expressed in bitter shredding adulations
Turned to wholly hollow Desecration
Despising when denied

Heavy shit ...Quit

I'm up again
Drowned on skies and clouded visions
Trying to disguise, with blurring lies, the confines of indecision
With selfish shrugs
And snorts of sniff
To eat away and
...A way further

Heavy shit...quit, quit, quit

Scrawl scratched blue
Into a bore
The score
Confessed of hope
Expressed in blank starring
An inertial resistance persisting
Past all caring
And that nothing thing
Happens

Pretending vainly the lies are true
I hide decried and desolate
Consoled within the shallow ending of the dream
The broken nightmare scream

Heavy shit gotta quit

But I ain't quit yet

The Long Night of the Urban Fox

The night burnt with its usual sodium glare
Restless in my bedroom
I envisioned that which was not there
Street light through the curtain
No longer left me certain
That the dark may be banished one more day
I lay starkly awake
Not convinced or ever since
That the shadows may not stay

The bed unhinged seemed made without comfort
No matter how the sheets were laid
Silence roared so loudly only to break like surf atop a wave
With bin lids rattling upon the pave outside
And in
I cringed to think
One day I might not be saved
That was not last time I would pray.
I felt in someway bitterly betrayed

Then a fox howled in a banshee's way
Its bark became a mocking bray
This is what I heard it say

"I'll follow you from here on in
Step your steps until you begin
To unsee me stalk around your mind
You will feed me with your future
Know your life is mine
Your brooding blood's the wine
I will drink as I dine upon your flesh
Our fates are now forever meshed
I'll lurk until your breath
Is rank with the sweet stink of death"

The vulpine scream had turned me white
Then the fox skulked from the orange light
Off to follow some secret rite
And I could never sleep as tightly
As I had before
That long night of the urban fox
Would leave me
                    Nevermore

The Slut I Am

Yes, I am
A slut
    I put out
            Easy
Feed me...
    Drinky
                Lead me
       By
    My pinkie
       And I will
            Follow
Then give it...
    Freely...

But I feel...
         ...Or used to

        (Though so long ago
        It's hard to know)

When I imagined
With, youthful sentiment
       How my life would lead
       That I would give
And in the act
Of giving
Would be freed

           But the truth

  Is so, so sleazy

  And that is why

I
    Am
       Soooo!
         ...Easy

The impotence of being ...Earnest

The Ballad of Ernie Burns

The early bird
Catches a word
Which then
Passes through
Its digestive tract

And some many years before
A terrible fate befell
Our erstwhile zero
Bleary-eyed hero
Ernie
...He was born
Which went on to became a thorn
To tear a world in two
Ripping it grey
Producing double visions
Of religious significance
At least, as spiritually corrupt
As all possession without touch
The colour rush explosions
Leathern skin
Tanned hide
Trailing thoughts
Behind his iron blood
Congealed and crusted
In oxides
Eating them
Growing fat
On oxygen
Consuming the composite element of burning
Infused with dreams
Of demons guzzling his dreams

The process he adopted
Was the way pomegranates follow
To grow albino
And blind to every winter
Attempting to die in stories
So they can live
Forever, also
The epigram finally true

"Ernie Burns cannot die
He can only have his character assassinated"

So, he drank another and another
Then designated his craziness driver
And let it cruise
A destructive path

The impotence of being ...Earnest

It is mighty so it's right all righty
No matter, the wrongs
He omits or admits
What is lacked in fine rhetoric and wit
Is made up for in copious dollops
Of steaming bullshit

So, that was the Ballad of E B Burns
The moral being:
Watch your back
'Cos they are taking it in turns

<u>The Karma Police</u>

I suffered an injustice
So, I called the Karma police
And after consulting with their records

They told me they were pleased
To inform me after all they had observed

They believed I had received
Just what I had deserved

Broker than Broken

The pub closes
And the last few
Wobble through doors
Home
Towards the boxes
They shelter their worlds inside
From the world out

Rank puddles of other's expectations
Drench our unwashed feet
Through pickled shoes

And before shutting up
We catch a moment
I offer you a cigarette
Or a chance to escape
You take neither
Cherishing restraint
Like a gifted favour from a lover
                        Would be treasured

Maybe in duty to the northern hemisphere
The attitude
That you have adopted in exile in London
Over the years
You no longer smile as you work

And I watch and wonder why
No one has rescued you

Flying the Desk

The educator cum aviator
Caused a murmur from his students
Who had noticed his empty stare
The sideways glance
Down the grained desk
As if it were
Speckled with darker seams
Beneath the veneer shine
Worn to an unbelievable smoothness
…Like sky
The green waste bin below
The green should be fields
The wood living trees
And three hundred feet below

Then a pupil interrupted

"'Scuse me sir!
You were talking
'Bout that Greek designer bloke
Before you blacked out…
You were talking some shit
About him, using wax and feathers
…To fly?
Forget it…
It just wouldn't have worked
It would have just broke in pieces
Like them fools in chicken suits
Jump off piers at Easter"

The teacher regarded the child
"It was because he did not listen
That Icarus was lost
Maybe you could learn a lesson from him?
No?
Now turn the page
And read to the end of the chapter"

But like orgasms and car crashes
Flash into the mind
The master was recaptured
In the mirage space between
Where gravity had taken him
And what the air loved to indulge
His chair squeaked
As his bird nature
Longing for its home in breezes and soaring
Made his arms stretch wide
Then swoop side to side

The impotence of being ...Earnest

The kids sniggered
But it did not break the far off look
In his glazed eyes
Skies reflected in his glasses
The desk flown into his mind of horizons
Escaping his capture in
A labyrinth of his own creation
"Daedlus made it out"
He thought
"But at what cost?
What had he lost?
Was it worth it?"

Robot Ballerina Dancing
In the Stars

Her dance resonates to rhythms only the skies observe
Night is for her to weave through
And let weave through her
Obscured by it veiling sullen dark
Her beauty scar is hidden
For the reason...
That light instead of blood had spilled
When the cut had left its mark
...Half over healed now
Where her parents had explained, had told her
She had fallen from a chair
With no word of the brightness pouring from the wound
And the doctors had in response
Had replaced her flesh with plates of metal skin
That would reflect inwardly the outward rays of sun star shine
So she could talk to them
Recall was she was
And be protected from the vacuum
The doctors knew she would endeavour to attain
She was space dust after all
They knew she would try to find succour there
The tutu was her own idea it would identify her as an artist
And so, she dances now
 In the stars
She is space dust after all

Untitled
(Stupid words)

We misspoke earlier
We said the end was nigh
When it had already happened
Therefore we misspoke
We were not involved earlier
in the flood we stood on the dead
We kept our heads
So we were not involved
We did not determine the outcome
We were only spectators
Eyes closed
Screwed tightly to avoid the truth
Grimly determined

We were misunderstood earlier
"They" jumped to conclusions
But the end had already happened
So we were misunderstood

Now we must move on